ATKINS DIET
The Ultimate Weight Loss Guide, with Low-Carb and Healthy Tips

Table of Contents

Introduction

There are many different diets out there but there aren't many diets that are quite as unique or useful for your life as the Atkins diet. This is a diet that will certainly change your life.

This book will help you understand everything that comes about when you're aiming to find a way to lose weight. This is a solution that can help you with losing a large amount of weight in particular.

This can be perfect if you have a large amount of weight to lose. This can be ideal if you have 40 pounds or more of weight to lose as there is no limit on what you can lose on the Atkins diet.

By using the Atkins diet, you will easily burn off fats as your body becomes used to burning them in lieu of carbohydrates. This works with a process known as ketosis.

This low-carb diet option works with an extensive variety of great foods. You will learn all about the many great foods that come with this diet plan throughout the book. Information on what to avoid or to at least be cautious around will also be covered in this book.

The details that are included around this book are very extensive and can certainly make a difference in your life. You will certainly benefit from the Atkins diet when it is used properly and with enough care.

Chapter 1 – A Basic Understanding of the Atkins Diet

The Atkins diet has been a very popular dietary choice for generations. This comes as it is a diet that is easy to follow with a simple concept.

The Atkins diet works as a diet where you consume lower amounts of carbohydrates while adding more protein and fat into your diet. This is a simple dietary plan but it is one that will certainly be effective when used right.

The diet focuses heavily on improving how ketosis works in the body. This works as fats stored within the body are burned off as energy.

The concept is to keep the body from taking in more glucose than needed. This includes the glucose that comes from carbohydrates. As this diet works, the participant will start to burn off fat as energy instead of the carbs that come in one's diet.

This is a unique dietary solution that can work over time. It is not as difficult for you to maintain as you might expect either.

A History of the Diet

The Atkins diet is a special concept that has been around for more than fifty years. The diet is named after Robert Atkins, a cardiologist who developed the process based on how he lost weight.

In 1963, Atkins had gained a large amount of weight and wanted to find a diet that could help him. It was then that he read a medical journal entry from Dr. Alfred Pennington on weight loss.

Pennington's work suggested that a restrictive diet can be used to treat obesity. In particular, an increase in fats and proteins and a reduction of sugar and carbohydrates in one's diet should be used to improve how well the body can lose weight.

Atkins tried this out and found it to be especially useful. He started to lose weight and began taking in a healthier lifestyle. Over time, he promoted his diet plan to more people and even got you work published in Vogue magazine.

Over the years Atkins continued to grow his business upon his diet by focusing on the results that come from it. He formed Atkins Nutritionals in 1998 as a company that consults people looking to lose weight and offers various low-carb and high-protein foods for consumption.

Over the years the Atkins diet has been a trusted option for all those looking to lose weight. Today you might find plenty of Atkins-branded products out on the market. Some restaurant chains have even gone so far as to serve Atkins-friendly products. Still, you can easily use the diet based on your needs.

The diet has become especially trustworthy in recent years. With more than seventy clinical studies out there proving that this diet works, this is a solution that will certainly work wonders for your life.

A Basic Consideration

The key consideration for the Atkins diet is that it focuses on keeping your blood sugar levels steady. As you consume carbohydrates, your body will start to experience up and down sugar levels. This causes you to store fats as you are using those carbs for energy.

Meanwhile, the Atkins diet will help you keep your blood sugar levels steady. This allows you to start burning off fats as you will be more controlled in terms of your blood sugar. As a result, your body will store less fat.

The Atkins diet can also keep you from experiencing feelings of hunger or sudden cravings for various foods. This prevents overeating, a common cause of excess weight gain.

It is true that more calories are consumed on this diet when compared with others, what with the added fats involved. These will provide you with more energy during the day. This in turn keeps you from being hungry. Simply put, you will actually feel full and lose weight during the day.

By using this diet, you will experience a substantial change in your body. You will start to burn off fat as you will keep your carb intake under control. As a result, it should be very easy for you to stay healthy and protected.

Chapter 2 – What Makes the Atkins Diet Perfect?

The Atkins diet certainly sounds like a great idea. The truth is that it is more advantageous than many other diets out there. In fact, the Atkins diet has plenty of advantages over many other traditional diets that you might have tried in the past.

Ketosis Is the Key

The main point about the Atkins diet is that it will help promote the process of ketosis. This is the key aspect of burning fat that must work.

Normally, your body will burn off the carbohydrates that you take in above everything else. This is a real problem when today's diets are concerned. We eat so many foods with carbs these days that we end up taking in more than necessary, thus keeping us from actually burning off fats.

When the body doesn't have lots of carbs, it will start to use fats for energy. This is the main focus of the Atkins diet.

Ketosis occurs when your body stops burning off carbohydrates and starts to burn fats. This works as the body does not have enough carbs to work with. As the body has fewer carbs, its blood sugar level will become stable. This allows the body to burn off fats as it will be less likely to store those fats.

The fats that are burned off will provide the body with the energy it requires. This can especially work well when the body takes in enough calories in one's diet.

By having a diet with plenty of fat and protein, your body will trigger ketosis. This comes as you will have fewer carbs and a newer form of energy to burn off. As your body burns off the fat, the items you consume and the fats that have been stored in your body from earlier will be burned off properly. This in turn improves how well your body can stay healthy. Ketosis can work for as long as needed. The goal is to take the fats in your body and to burn them off the right way. This will really make a difference when you are aiming to stay healthy.

As you stay with the Atkins diet, ketosis will continue to work well enough to keep your body from adding more fat than needed. This can make a true difference when prepared right.

What Weight Loss Results Will You Get?

The weight loss that you will attain will vary based on how well you complete the diet and how long you use it for. There is a potential for you to lose a great deal of weight depending on how well this plan works.

You can lose about two pounds per week as you use the diet over time. This is a controlled amount of weight loss that should be easy for your body to handle.

You may experience a little more weight loss at the very start. In particular, you might lose about five to ten pounds in the first two to three weeks of the diet. This should encourage you to continue working with the diet as your body starts to feel better over time. This is beset used by those who have large amounts of weight that they need to burn off. People who are 40 or more pounds overweight can especially take advantage of this diet plan. There is another form of the Atkins diet for those who have less of a need to lose weight as you will learn in a future chapter.

Basic Benefits Outside Weight Loss

There are plenty of other great benefits that come outside weight loss:

- This may keep epilepsy from being a problem as it eases the symptoms of this condition.

- Acid reflux levels will be reduced in your body as you use the diet.

- Headaches will be less likely to occur. This can especially work wonders for those who experience migraine headaches.

- The diet reduces inflammation in the body and lowers one's blood pressure. This in turn reduces the body's risk of experiencing serious heart issues.

- The risk of dementia and other age-related mental disorders may be reduced while on the Atkins diet.

Why It's Better Than Other Options

The Atkins diet will especially be a smarter diet option when compared with other choices out there. It is better than diets that focus on carbs. These include the Paleo diet, a diet that takes a look at the quality of carbs but does not have limits on them. While the Paleo diet does entail healthy carbs from nuts and seeds, the diet does not have restrictions on how many can be used. The Atkins diet focuses on ensuring that the carbs one consumes are as minimal as possible while also focusing on healthy carb options.

In fact, the diet is certainly better than the Mediterranean diet as that option will cause you to become too dependent on carbohydrates. The Atkins diet helps you learn how to handle carbs the right way as you reduce your totals.

It is also easier for you to maintain the Atkins diet over time. The problem with many of the other diet options out there is that they can be difficult to handle as they often hold restrictions even greater than what the Atkins diet has. The Paleo diet, for instance, holds extreme limits on the fruits and vegetables you can have and obviously omits dairy. The food selections on the Atkins diet are clearly more diverse.

The Atkins diet will be an ideal option for your body. This is a great diet that should support your body and provide you with the assistance needed to keep your weight in check.

Chapter 3 – Starting With the Induction Phase

The Atkins diet works with four phases. These are designed to help you along the entire diet.

When used properly, the four phases will help you to not only start losing weight but to also improve how well your body can burn off fats. However, you must be careful when starting out the diet as it can be critical to your success.

The first phase of the Atkins diet is the induction phase. This lasts for about two weeks but it is clearly the most important phase in the entire diet.

The induction phase is used to introduce your body to the Atkins diet. That is, it is to get the body to start burning off fats through ketosis.

You must have 25 grams of carbs at the most. The substantial reduction in the total will certainly have to be considered.

This is done by heavily restricting the total number of carbs that you are going to consume in a typical day. You will have to consume more high-fat and high-protein foods with fewer carbs to make this work. In particular:

- Healthy fats from meats should be consumed.

- Most cheeses are acceptable at this point.

- Low-carb vegetables can always be used at this point.

The induction phase will keep your body from taking in more carbs. This in turn signals the body to start burning off fats. This process especially works as you consume enough calories and proteins to keep your body active and ready to lose weight.

As the fat-burning starts, your body will begin to be used to burn off fat instead of carbs. This comes as the total amount of fat in your body will be substantially reduced.

The induction phase is often considered by many to be the most difficult part of the process. This is due to how you will have to restrict the foods that you are eating. The substantial limits involved in the diet can be tough on some people but these limits can make a difference when used properly.

During the induction phase, you will have to avoid high-carb fruits and vegetables. You will especially have to omit all starches and legumes from your diet. These include beans, potatoes and many others. These may be added later on in your diet although it is best to keep them at minimal quantities if possible.

This is a process that may result in a little more weight loss than other parts. In particular, you may get close to five to ten pounds of fat off your body during these two weeks.

You can always stay in the induction phase for longer than two weeks if desired. However, the results may not be as consistent during the later weeks as what you might get at the start. The fact that this is a difficult stage to maintain for longer than two weeks will make this a challenge to handle.

A 14-Day Plan

You can easily take advantage of the induction phase with a sensible diet. This should work with the right types of foods to keep your body from taking in more carbs.

This 14-day plan is designed to help you with getting the most out of the induction phase. You can always substitute different meats at various points in this part of the diet but it helps to think carefully when looking to do things right.

As you will notice, much of this entails a good amount of meat each day. These meals should be consumed with enough fats and proteins from meats to get your body to adjust to a low-carb lifestyle.

Day 1
Breakfast: 1 egg
Lunch: 4 ounces salmon
Dinner: 6 ounces turkey
Snack: 1 dill pickle
Day 2
Breakfast: 4 ounces chicken
Lunch: 4 ounces tuna
Dinner: 5 ounces beef
Snack: 2 ounces celery with a dollop of heavy whipping cream
Day 3
Breakfast: 1 egg with 2 slices bacon
Lunch: 4 ounces chicken
Dinner: 6 ounces pork with one ounce lettuce
Snack: 1 broccoli stalk
Day 4
Breakfast: 3 slices bacon with 2 ounces lettuce
Lunch: 4 ounces veal with 2 ounces spinach

Dinner: 5 ounces cod with 1 celery stalk

Snack: 1 or 2 radishes

Day 5

Breakfast: 1 egg

Lunch: 5 ounces chicken

Dinner: 6 ounces uncured ham with half a cup turnip greens

Snack: 3 to 5 green olives

Day 6

Breakfast: 1 egg and 2 slices bacon

Lunch: 4 ounces lamb with one ounce broccoli

Dinner: 4 ounces crab meat

Snack: 1 celery stalk

Day 7

Breakfast: 2 ounces turkey sausage

Lunch: 4 ounces oysters

Dinner: 5 ounces lobster meat with 1 ounce cucumber slices

Snack: 1 diced bell pepper

Day 8

Breakfast: 3 ounces pork sausage

Lunch: 4 ounces beef with 1 ounce spinach

Dinner: 4 ounces chicken with 1 celery stalk

Snack: 1 ounce macadamia nuts

Day 9

Breakfast: 1 egg with 2 slices of bacon

Lunch: 4 ounces sardines with included oil

Dinner: 4 ounces herring with 1 ounce broccoli

Snack: 1 full pickle

Day 10

Breakfast: 4 ounces turkey sausage

Lunch: 3 ounces oysters with half a celery stalk

Dinner: 4 ounces veal and half a cup raw button mushrooms

Snack: Half an avocado

Day 11

Breakfast: 4 ounces pork sausage

Lunch: Half a cup cabbage with 4 ounces chicken

Dinner: 4 ounces turkey and 2 tablespoons leeks

Snack: Half a cup cooked collard greens

Day 12

Breakfast: 2 eggs

Lunch: 4 ounces turkey with 1 tablespoon minced garlic

Dinner: 4 ounces tuna with half a cup Brussel sprouts

Snack: 1 turnip

Day 13

Breakfast: 1 egg and 1 ounce gouda cheese

Lunch: 4 ounces spinach and half a diced cucumber

Dinner: 4 ounces beef with 1 tablespoon parmesan cheese

Snack: 1 celery stalk with 2 tablespoons of bleu cheese

Day 14

Breakfast: 2 slices bacon with 1 egg

Lunch: 4 ounces turkey with 2 ounces spinach

Dinner: 4 ounces beef with 1 ounce cabbage

Snack: Half an avocado

As you might notice through this guide, there are a few simple standards to use when eating during this part of the diet. You have to focus heavily on meats and vegetables to make this all work. You need plenty of food in each meal while also having a good snack to make it work right.

When you follow this part of the diet, you will become used to how it works and what you can get out of it. This can take a bit for you to complete but when done properly, it will be easier for you to feel healthy and capable.

Remember, the induction phase is clearly the toughest part of the Atkins diet because of how restrictive it is when compared with the other stages. It will truly be worth it when you consider how your body will respond to it. Just imagine how you will get on the path to losing weight the right way.

Chapter 4 – The Three Remaining Stages

After you are done with the induction stage of the Atkins diet, you can get to the next few stages. These are easier to handle, what with there being fewer restrictions involved at these points. Still, you have to be careful when consuming foods at these stages. These stages can last a little longer depending on how much weight you are trying to lose. The standards you have for losing weight will vary based on your personal needs but you should at least look carefully to see what you can get out of your diet at this point.

Balancing

After your body gets used to the Atkins diet, you will be able to add a few foods back into your diet. This occurs in the second stage, the balancing stage.
You can have from 25 to 50 grams or carbs each day. This is much more than what you had earlier but it is still minimal enough to where you will control the total amount of carbs that you are consuming.
During this stage, you will start to add nuts and seeds and some fruits and vegetables back into your diet. These should include low-carb fruits and vegetables for the most part.
The following foods are appropriate:
- All foods included in the induction stage

- Cherries, berries and other antioxidant-rich fruits

- Whole milk yogurt

- Legumes including lima beans, lentils and chickpeas

- Tomato, lemon and lime juices (only take a few tablespoons of lemon or lime juices each day)

This is to help you maintain a healthy balance in your body as you consume a healthy amount of carbs without going overboard. You will especially be eating healthier carbs.

The weight loss that comes from this stage can be for about one to three pounds of fat each week. This is a safe amount of weight loss in that your body can easily adjust to the losses.

This part of the diet can last for as long as needed. It can last for a few weeks depending on how much fat you are aiming to burn off. You will clearly need to spend more time with this if you have more fat to burn off.

Fine-Tuning

The third stage is the fine-tuning stage. This is a part where you can gradually added carbs into your body. The key is to let this work with a sensible total to allow the weight loss to continue. This is a point where you should lose about one pound of weight each week.

You, might have to reduce your carb total in the event that your weight loss stops or is dramatically reduced. Either way, you need about 50 to 80 grams of carbs at this point each day.

You should be cautious when increasing the grams you consume though. You can always add five to ten more grams of carbs each day so long as you stay within the proper limit used at this stage in the diet. The goal is for you to reach your targeted weight and to maintain it. This weight should be kept for about a month so your body will have an easier time handling it.

The various kinds of foods that were listed in the first two stages can be used at this point. You can add the following at this stage:

- Other added fruits may be included although you should be cautious so you don't have too many with lots of sugars. Cherries, apples, mangoes and bananas are always good to have.

- Starchy vegetables may be added although it helps to consume them in smaller quantities.

- Whole grains can be included like sorghum, barley and oats. Make sure these are not processed and that you consume them responsibly. Also, these grains should be cooked.

This part can work for as long as necessary. The goal is to simply see that you can get to your target weight and keep it there. You might end up losing a little more weight although it is best to stick to being around your targeted weight to make this diet work out right.

Maintenance

The last stage of the Atkins diet is the maintenance stage. This is an ongoing phase that will entail maintaining your new healthy weight. This helps you to keep a healthy weight without adding more food into your diet than necessary. This is a very sensible and useful part of the diet that ensures that you will have enough food to consume without going overboard.

This is a great part of the Atkins diet that will entail about 50 to 130 carbs each day. This should be enough to provide you with energy but low enough to where your body will still work hard enough to burn off fats.

The points that you must follow while on the Atkins diet can make a difference in terms of how successful it can be. You must make sure the right parts of the diet are followed so it will be easier for you to lose weight and keep it offer properly. This will certainly make a difference when handled carefully enough.

Chapter 5 – Critical Nutrients

There are plenty of nutrients that are essential to the Atkins diet. While you need to consume more fats and proteins and fewer carbs, there are many other things that have to be added to your diet just as well. Many of these nutrients can be added to your diet through the foods that you consume. These will be essential for making it easier for your body to handle the diet the right way.

Omega-3 Fatty Acids

You must have omega-3 fatty acids in your diet so it will stay healthy. These are fats that help to improve how blood flows around your body. This in turn makes it easier for your body to stay healthy. Omega-3 fatty acids are capable of reducing inflammation around your body. This is especially the case in your arteries as it improves how well blood will flow over time.

In addition, these fatty acids will improve upon the HDL cholesterol levels in your body. These levels will increase over time as you take in enough omega-3 fats. This should improve how blood flows and can improve how blood cells move without sticking together or being misshapen.

It is critical to have omega-3 fatty acids in your Atkins diet plan as the human body cannot produce this fat on its own. Fortunately, many of the fish products you can consume while on the Atkins diet will certainly help you out. In fact, the oils that come from fish – or fish oil as it is called – contain plenty of omega-3s.

Iron

You will need plenty of iron for energy. Iron improves how red blood cells are formed in your body. As they are formed properly, your body will become energetic as it will be easier for nutrients to move around your body.
Iron can particularly be found in many meats. This is especially the case with beef. Adding enough iron to your diet will help you stay active and ready for anything during the day.

Fiber

Fiber can be found in a variety of green vegetables in the Atkins diet. While it is true that fiber is often associated with grains, the truth is that you don't need lots of grains with carbs to get fiber. Green vegetables can always help you out with your fiber. This is especially the case with spinach, one of the best high-fiber vegetables around.

Fiber is critical as it improves how well your body handles its blood sugar levels. It keeps blood sugar levels consistent for a longer period of time. This ensures that your body can continue to burn off fats. This should be easier for the body to handle when used properly enough.

Antioxidants

Antioxidants are important to your body in that they will control the development of unhealthy toxins and free radicals. These are compounds that can build up in your body as a result of an unhealthy diet. These may also come about as a result of the many toxins that pollute our environment.
Antioxidants are used to bind to these free radicals. These will neutralize them and all these to be removed naturally throughout the entire body. This should make it easier for the body to recover and stay healthy.

Chapter 6 – A Lighter Version of the Atkins Diet

The Atkins diet is clearly a challenge for many but it can be advantageous and useful if you manage it properly. There are a few things to consider when trying to make the Atkins diet work right for your needs.

This chapter features a lighter option to consider when trying to make the Atkins diet work for you. This can help you out quite well if you need some help with getting through the diet

This lighter version is especially perfect for when you are trying to prepare for the induction phase. This helps you get a clear idea of what foods you can have during the Atkins diet. While the induction phase is still substantially restricted when compared with this, you will at least start out with a smarter version of the diet.

40 Grams Is the Key

The key part of this option is to consume 40 grams of carbohydrates in a day. This should be divided up as evenly as possible between three meals and two snacks.

You can always add 10 grams of carbs each day when you get a little closer to your targeted weight goal. Try to avoid consuming more than 70 grams of carbs for the best results.

Foods To Have

This works with three four to six-ounce servings of protein in a day with two to four servings of fats. These should be balanced out well during the day. The proteins that you consume should be of any kind of meat that is acceptable on the diet. You can have various fish, chicken and beef items in particular. Eggs can also be included as part of the diet if desired.

For the added fats, about one tablespoon of butter, healthy oil or other acceptable fats may be included in three servings.

About 15 grams of carbs can be consumed in the vegetables you consume. Try and get about four to eight servings of vegetables each day for the best results.

The other 25 grams for the diet should be consumed with enough servings of other foods that can be accepted during the day. These include various nuts, healthy fruits and whole grains.

This lighter option may be useful if you need assistance with starting the Atkins diet. Be sure to think about this when looking for a simple and sensible way to start losing weight.

Chapter 7 – Foods to Eat

A great part of the Atkins diet is that there are plenty of great foods that you can eat. However, there are a few different foods that you must avoid, as you will discover later in this chapter.

The key about the Atkins diet is to consume the right fats and proteins. This is to help you get the energy you need as you can burn off the fats over time. This certainly works well as you will start to get your body to consume fewer carbs, thus making it easier for you to break down more fats.

Meats

There are plenty of great meats to have while on the Atkins diet. These include chicken, beef, pork and lamb among many others.

These meats work particularly well when prepared right. Many of these meats can be grilled or broiled in many cases. Also, lean cuts of these meats may be used if desired.

You should not be concerned about the fats that come with these meats as these will be burned off while on the diet. This should be easier for your body to process when used right.

Of course, you should avoid anything that contains trans fats or saturated fats. These facts are typically more likely to harm your body and are often harder to burn off. This is especially the case with trans fats although it is not too hard for saturated fats to be burned off if necessary.

Fish and Seafood

Fatty fish and seafood items are always great to have as they contain enough protein for your body to handle. Fatty fish especially contain omega-3 fatty acids, compounds that will help improve circulation in your body and reduce inflammation.

The types of fish and seafood products for you to consume should include options like salmon, trout, haddock and much more. The key is to look for fish that are properly prepared and cleaned.

The oils that come from these fish are especially important. These oils typically contain the highest concentrations of omega-3 fats and therefore should be used the most. By using them properly, it should be very easy for you to stay healthy without adding more stress to your body than necessary.

You should still be cautious when it comes to how much fish you consume. Some fish may contain mercury deposits. While these deposits are relatively minimal, you should at least pace yourself when consuming fish so you don't take in more mercury at a time than necessary.

Eggs

Eggs are very popular on the Atkins diet for how they contain plenty of healthy fats and proteins. Eggs can especially be consumed for breakfast or mixed in with assorted meats.

You can always have whole eggs or egg whites depending on your preference. You can also find omega-3 enriched eggs that will provide you this ideal fat for your body.

Eggs can be prepared in the following ways:

- Fried

- Scrambled

- Hard-boiled

- Soft-boiled

- Deilved

- Poached

These can be prepared with many healthy vegetables in omelets and can also be consumed alongside various meats. You can prepare these with all kinds of items so long as you consume them with enough fat and protein to support the diet.

Low-Carb Vegetables

While it is true that vegetables are certainly healthy and easy to consume, you should be cautious. Not all vegetables are appropriate for the Atkins diet as they might contain too many carbs. You will learn about those later in this book.

There are plenty of low-carb vegetables that will be easy for your diet. These include such great vegetables as the following:

- Various greens; these include lettuce and spinach

- Celery

- Radishes

- Mushrooms

- Asparagus

- Okra

- Avocado

- Cucumber

- Assorted peppers; jalapeno and green bell peppers are especially ideal

- Zucchini

- Broccoli

These are all vegetables that do not contain high starch totals. Therefore, they should be easy for you to consume in your regular diet.

Full-Fat Dairy

You have to consume full-fat dairy products in order to stay healthy. Great full-fat dairy products are ideal for how they add protein to your body and include enough fats for you to use as energy.
You should look for plenty of full-fat items like butter, cheese, yogurt and cream to help your body. These should be full-fat options as the skim options are not going to provide you with the necessary proteins needed to keep the diet going.

Nuts and Seeds

You can always use nuts and seeds when getting the Atkins diet to work right. These are products that contain various healthy fats and protein. The fats include monounsaturated fats that will control inflammation and improve how well blood flows in your body over time.

These are all ideal to have but they do contain some carbs. As a result, you must make sure you consume them with plenty of control. These are healthy carbs when compared to many others thanks to their fat contents but the key is to use these nuts and seeds responsibly. You don't want to consume more than what you should handle.

The best nuts and seeds to consume include almonds, walnuts, sunflower seeds and macadamia nuts. These typically have fewer carbs than many other nuts and seeds although it still helps to watch for how many of them you consume at a time.

Oils

Oils that come from foods are typically pressed. That is, they will come from foods as they are properly squeezed. The moisture contents from these foods will come out as oils that can be used on many foods. They are typically added as dressings but sometimes foods may be cooked in them to add a bit of extra flavor.

There are all kinds of great oils that can be added to your diet. These include coconut oil, avocado oil and extra virgin olive oil.

These oils may be added to all sorts of foods during the cooking process. These oils typically contain more healthy fats with omega-3 fatty acids especially being commonplace in many of them.

You should avoid oils that come from vegetables though. These oils tend to come from vegetables that are actually harmful to the Atkins diet.

Drinks To Have

Of course, you will need plenty of healthy drinks to make the Atkins diet easier on your body. There are plenty of good options to have:

- Water is clearly a necessity, what with how it keeps you hydrated and may also control your appetite. You should aim for at least eight 8-ounce glasses of water each day.

- Coffee contains antioxidants that will help to clear out old waste materials in your body. You can always add a full-fat creamer to your coffee as well. Make sure you avoid adding sugar though.

- Green tea is very popular for offering antioxidants as well. This also contains very few sugars.

- Alcohol can be consumed in small quantities if you have low-carb and low-sugar options. Dry wines that do not have any added sugars can always be ideal, for instance.

- Tomato juice is suitable after the induction phase is over.

Be sure to consume enough healthy drinks that are safe for your body. These should work well provided that you take in options that have fewer or no carbs or sugars.

Surprisingly Appealing Foods

One of the toughest parts of any diet, even one that offers many food options like the Atkins diet, is that they often don't have many foods that you might think are exciting. However, this is certainly not the case with the Atkins diet. The truth is that you can enjoy a few special treats here and there.
There are a few foods that are acceptable on the Atkins diet that are actually a little more indulgent, for lack of a better word. However, they are great to have during the diet. These are options that should be had in smaller quantities for the most part but they can still be useful.

- Nut butters like almond butter and walnut butter are great to have on lots of things. Your butters should be made with the nuts and salt without any outside added materials though.

- Dark chocolate contains plenty of fiber and antioxidants. This may also reduce your blood pressure. This type of chocolate is one that is not heavily processed and has a higher cocoa content with less sugar. Dark chocolate contains fewer carbs than other options but make sure the cocoa content is strong.

- Pork rinds are made with more protein. These contain monounsaturated fats and do not contain any carbs. Still, these contain omega-6 fatty acids that might wear out your arteries so it helps to be careful when eating them.

- Bacon is a very popular food product these days and is also a suitable thing to have on the Atkins diet. Most bacon fat is unsaturated so it will provide you with enough fat for your needs without being too harmful. However, you should look for nitrate-free bacon that has not been as heavily processed.

- Beef jerky can be great if you find a choice that has no added sugars or preservatives. You might have to get your own food dehydrator to make your own jerky though as many commercial options tend to use sugars and other items to keep their meats ready for consumption.

If anything, this listing of foods to have on the Atkins diet proves that this is a diet option that will certainly help your body. Still, as you will see in the next chapter, there are plenty of concerning points that need to be explored just as well.

Chapter 8 – Cautions For Foods

There are plenty of added considerations that must be used in your diet. This chapter is about understanding how certain foods may work if you are responsible enough with them. That is, there are some foods that should be avoided as well as ones that might be dangerous if you don't consume them the right way.

Foods to Avoid

There are plenty of harmful foods that will not do anything good for your Atkins diet needs. These are dangerous foods that can do more to impact your body in a negative way.

The key is to ensure you avoid consuming these foods:

- Sugars from soft drinks, pastries, candies and other items should be avoided.

- Processed grains like rice, wheat, rye and others must not be consumed. These contain more carbs than many other foods.

- Vegetable oils like corn and soybean oils should not be used.

- Trans fats are not healthy fats in that they increase inflammation and reduce circulation. These should always be avoided. These can be found in processed foods and anything that has been hydrogenated.

- Foods that claim to be diet or low-fat versions of foods should be avoided for how they contain more sugars. These added sugars are typically included to improve the textures of foods to keep them together.

Vegetables To Be Cautious Around

There are a number of vegetables that can be dangerous to the Atkins diet. These are vegetables that contain more starches. These are compounds that contain more carbs and as a result should be avoided in your diet for the best possible results. The vegetables that you need to avoid in your diet include the following problematic concerns:

- Peas

- Beets

- Potatoes; these include sweet potatoes

- Corn

- Water chestnuts

- Winter squashes, particularly butternut and acorn squashes

- Parsnips

Carrots are a unique consideration in this category. While it is true that carrots are a starch, they do not contain anywhere near as many carbs as other vegetables with starches. Therefore, you have to be cautious when adding carrots to your diet.

You can always add these vegetables during the last stage of the Atkins diet. These should still be avoided during the earliest stages though.

What About Fruits?

Fruits are known to contain sugars for the most part. Therefore, they are to be avoided during the induction phase of the diet. However, it will be easier for you to consume fruits when you are out of the induction phase.

Fruits are clearly designed for later stages of the diet as they contain more sugars. While these sugars are typically easier for the body to process, you should still be careful when having them.

The best fruits to have in your Atkins diet include these options that contain more antioxidants and fewer carbs:

- Berries, particularly strawberries, raspberries and blackberries

- Cantaloupe

- Honeydew

- Cherries

- Apples

- Watermelon

Consuming Healthy Grains

While it is true that many grains are dangerous and filled with lots of carbs that does not mean every grain in the world is bad. In particular, whole grains are easier for your body to have than others.
Whole grains are made from many sources including sorghum and millet. These are grains that are not processed and contain more fiber. They are slower for the body to digest, thus controlling your appetite and keeping your blood sugar levels under control. You should consider whole grains like oat bran, polenta, steel-cut oats and buckwheat among other healthy grains. Of course, you have to be cautious with these grains as you still need to consume enough to stay within your limit. Of course, these grains will not be appropriate during the earliest stages of the diet.

A Word on Alcohol

Alcohol can be consumed if desired but you have to think carefully about what you're consuming. You can always have one drink of alcohol each day or every other day. You can always consider a simple drink to be a little reward.
However, that does not mean you can have any kind of alcohol. You have to be a little more controlled when consuming alcohol.

Here are a few options to have:

- Most beer contains plenty of carbs but some light options will contain 5 or fewer carbs in each 12-ounce serving.

- Many types of wine will contain fewer carbs. A glass of red or white wine will contain about 2 grams of carbs. Dry wine will contain even fewer carbs. Dessert wines and other wines with sugar should be avoided.

- Pure spirits contain little to no carbs on average. These include whiskey, vodka and brandy.

- Use soda water and lime when trying to mix a drink. These do not contain any carbs. Anything that is too sugary can be harmful; a White Russian has about 20 grams of carbs per serving, for instance.

The most important thing to do when consuming alcohol is to be extremely cautious. It is easier for the body to become intoxicated when one consumes too much alcohol during a low carb diet. Much of this could be due to the liver working hard to process the fats that you take in.

Chapter 9 – Can a Vegetarian Handle the Atkins Diet?

It's clear that meat is a crucial part of the Atkins diet. It is needed so you can get the protein and fat necessary for the diet.

This leaves a big question on the table – what if you are trying to live with a vegetarian lifestyle?

The fact is that you can actually use the Atkins diet if you are a vegetarian. There are plenty of good vegetables to use as you read earlier. Great plant-based fat sources like olive and coconut oils can always be good for your body. The right nuts and seeds will especially be important for your life.

You can always have plenty of dairy products in your diet if you are willing to use them. Some vegetarians will consume dairy products and eggs although others will not. Still, these are available for your use. Full-fat dairy products are clearly required.

In terms of replacing the meat on the Atkins diet, you can always use soy-based foods. Soy has long been used as a substitute for meat products. This is thanks to how soy can be prepared in enough shapes that are similar to other meats.

More importantly, soy contains plenty of fat and protein. This may be comparable with other meats in your diet. Therefore, soy can certainly work well during the diet.

If anything, the Atkins diet may require some sacrifices among those who are looking to live with vegetarian diets. This comes from how tough it might be to have it without consuming any meats. Be sure to think about this and plan your dietary needs ahead of time by considering the particular vegetables you need or whatever soy items you want to consume.

Remember, it might be a little harder for the Atkins diet to work if you are trying to use a vegetarian diet. This could still help you out if used properly and with enough care.

Chapter 10 – What Side Effects Can Occur?

While the Atkins diet can be ideal, there are a few side effects that may occur as a result. These are relatively minimal and are more likely to develop during the earlier induction stage. As you go through with the diet, you will become less likely to suffer from many of these problems. Even so, you should at least be aware of what may come about when you are aiming to make the diet work for you.

What Ketosis Causes

The ketosis process, as beneficial as it is, will cause a few side effects. These problems include the following issues:

- Bad breath

- Fatigue

- Dizziness

- Nausea

- Insomnia

These effects will occur at the start of ketosis and will be less intense as you become used to your diet. The added proteins in your diet should help you with getting enough energy to counter the fatigue you might experience in the diet.

Early Bowel Discomfort

As you start the Atkins diet, you might experience a bit of discomfort in your bowels. This comes as you are starting to clear out more waste materials from your body.

Much of this is thanks to how you are starting to clear out fats from your body. The burning of fats can cause the amount of waste you have to expel to become larger after a while. This might cause your bowel movements to be hard to handle at the start.

However, the risk of bowel discomfort will be reduced as you get used to the Atkins diet. As your body begins to lose weight in a controlled manner, you will find your bowel movements to be a little easier to handle than you might expect.

This discomfort might be a challenge but no matter what happens, you should not try to take any medicines to ease the issue. The problem with some laxatives or softeners is that they might add more fatigue onto your bowels than necessary. They might cause some parts of your bowels to weaken and wear out.

Heart Issues From the Wrong Fats

You must be very cautious when consuming the fats that you take in your diet. While fats are important to the diet, you have to avoid taking in fats that might be too dangerous to your body.

Specifically, trans fats and an extreme amount of saturated fats can cause fatigue on your heart and your arteries. This could keep you from staying healthy.

Always check on the fat contents that come with your foods. The best fats are natural ones that come directly from the animal or egg among other sources. Anything that has omega-3 fatty acids will certainly be perfect as mentioned earlier.

Be sure to watch how you use the Atkins diet. The diet can cause some side effects although most of them are at the start. Some of these effects can be prevented too.

Chapter 11 – Tips For Success

To make the Atkins diet work for you, it helps to take a closer look at some of the many things you can do to make your body healthy.

Consider Your Portions

Make sure you think carefully about the portions you plan on consuming when following the Atkins diet. You have to avoid having portions that are too large. In particular, having four to six ounces of food at each meal should be good enough.

This encourages you to have a healthy amount of food without being too hard to follow. This can particularly encourage you to get the most out of your routine.

This can especially be sensible when you are out of the house and eating. You should try and aim to get smaller portions if possible so you at least keep the possible carb intake of whatever you are having under control.

Plan Ahead

It's always a good idea to plan your meals ahead of time. A great diet can entail meals that you know are appropriate and carefully laid out. This should help you with keeping yourself healthy.

You must especially determine what you plan on eating before you shop for groceries. This is to ensure that you don't get back into any old habits that you might have had.

Consider Eating Out On Occasion

As great as it is for you to easily consume a variety of healthy foods at home, you can always consider going out to eat on occasion. This can be perfect if you just want to enjoy something for the night.

You can always eat out for fun but you should at least look at the options that are at the place you want to visit. While many different restaurants have prepared a variety of great low-carb options, you have to do your research. You might be surprised at home many places are willing to omit breads and other carbs from recipes on request.

You must still watch for how foods are prepared at any place that you might want to dine out at. While the farm to table movement has been prominent in recent time as organic farming has been a hit at many restaurants, that doesn't mean every place is safe. You have to look carefully at whatever it is you want to consume so you will have a healthy option without worrying about how the foods were made.

Naturally, it is often easier for you to get a salad at one of these places that you can eat out at. There are plenty of other things you can do with regards to eating out:

- See if you can get lettuce instead of bread for your meal. This is ideal for burgers, tacos and other items that typically use breads.

- A bowl option can be great for things like tacos, burritos and other items that can be mixed together.

- Avoid things that are battered or sweetened. Many batters are used to add flavors to a meat or to keep the meat together but they are not necessary.

- Pizza can be useful provided you load up enough toppings and avoid consuming the crust if possible. A knife and fork can help you out to keep from eating much of the crust on your pizza. On a related note, look for the thinnest possible pizza option so you can avoid having too many carbs.

Conclusion

As you have discovered throughout this entire book, the Atkins diet is certainly an option for your body that will make a real difference. The Atkins diet will be easy for you to handle when you understand the proper foods to have.

This diet works with an extensive variety of great foods that are easy for you to consume. They will certainly work wonders for your body as they will help you burn off fat.

This diet can last for a long time so long as you put in the right effort. This will lead you to a healthier lifestyle that is easier to handle. Best of all, there should be no limit as to how much fat you can burn off with this option.

Good luck in your effort to complete the Atkins diet. You will certainly be proud of yourself when you see just how better and healthier your body is when you use this diet to your advantage.